©2011Michaeldawson
Lite Version

I0428686

COPYRIGHT

12 Fat Ladies

By Michael Dawson

Lite version 8.0

Licence

This book remains the copyright of its author at all times. (c) Michael Dawson 2010. It is for the reader and owner to experience and may not be copied or shared without the authors permission. All rights are reserved under the law of the country of purchase. The book is produced for your own enjoyment and interest with advice given in the very best spirit. The author accepts no responsibility whatsoever for claims made in relation to its content and outside his control. How the work is used remains the readers full responsibility and discression.

INTRODUCTION

Being on a diet makes you fat and is bad for your health. The evidence shows that in general your diet will be an indicator of weight GAIN! You are probably aware on a personal level that there is no need for any long term in depth study to determine this because its likely your experience bears this out. Over years of different schemes and false dawns its likely you have gained weight overall. If this is true then the cruel truth is that you may have followed the mantra that it is all your fault. On the front page of diet monthly you have seen the super slimmers and the weightless and said "if only I had the willpower to do that" and believed it was true. You may never have considered that it was the fault of the diet itself. Not just the diet in particular but the very fact that you are on one in the first place. Because being on a diet makes you do the very opposite of what you should be doing. I want to try and explain why this is true and argue that the only way forward is to give up diets forever. To make small long lasting changes at the right mental level and start to enjoy your life without the constant message that it was you that failed again when in fact failure was inevitable. Once the diet is gone then we can work on replacing it with something that works on a much higher level and is better for your health and wellbeing.

Mankind is in a unique position right now, one which they have never before encountered since the beginning of time. Affluence and better standards of living are reaching a bigger part of a growing global population. Most developed societies are fine-tuned to provide everything we need to eat and survive whilst exercise has become choice not necessity. As a result the population of the world gets bigger in more ways than one as life becomes easier and natural diets change. Our bodies are designed to be physically active beings who seek out food when we can and store it within our bodies as fat for leaner times. The problem is spreading across the developed world and so is the demand for an answer to mass obesity. As our society has struggled with the problem we spend billions of pounds looking for it. From pills to potions to miracle diets and weight loss schemes we spend billions every year. The diet industry is king and we are all under its spell. In the meantime if what they offer doesn't work, they make you believe it's your fault not theirs.

The whole world is under the spell of the diet industry which claims to offer hope in many guises to people who are suffering. They offer a chance to beat the weight, become slim and beautiful again. A chance to live in a world where you will be active, fit and happy. Like a strange cult they offer hope but sadly the evidence shows that's all they offer, just hope. In a UCLA study of thirty or more other studies combined the author Traci Mann said her research suggested that the very fact you were on a diet was an indicator of weight gain! That's right, being on a diet is an indicator of WEIGHT GAIN!

Mann Said "The benefits of dieting are too small and the potential harm too large for dieting to be recommended as a safe effective treatment of obesity"

This kind of research fails to alter the magic of the diet industry unless you are one of it's clients that is. Even the mother of one of the researchers said "what they are saying is obvious" after yo- yo dieting for years.

The business offers a myriad of diet schemes from colour codes to calorie counting from points systems to food parcels. We know it doesn't work because the evidence clearly shows that. I don't mean it does not work for you I mean it does not work at all. In fact one study showed that it was as good as doing nothing at all.

"Sure it does" I hear you say " I saw that woman who was slimmer of the year and she looked great" Hey listen I heard of a guy smoked 10 packs a day and lived to be 95 does that mean smoking is good for you?

Dieting is like some kind of global cult but it doesn't just affect small groups of people it affects billions of people. Even those who are not overweight believe that the best way of losing weight is to diet. People have become enslaved for entire lifetimes battling against their weight using the very thing that keeps them big. That's right, diets will make you bigger and more dependent in the long run. It's a multi-billion pound industry that is worshipped by all and questioned by few. They have convinced millions that they "need" food management. This unconscious conspiracy works in a similar way to any cult.

Like any cult they convince followers of a twisted reality using peer pressure and advertising. They create a belief system that is gospel and unquestionable. They preach that weight loss through diets is a real concept and the only way, if the diet fails then its your fault not theirs. Like a cult they make increasing demands upon us both physically and mentally. We are forced to suspend belief in the natural world and pay for miracle drugs, berries or tablets that will make a difference to our weight. The industry ignores any idea of rapid weight loss being bad for your health. Even though evidence suggests yo yo dieting could be linked to numerous health problems including altered immune function, stroke and diabetes. In the meantime the burden on our self-esteem brought about by their failure is carried on through life. Their leaders will spread stories of greatness to enhance their reputation with awards and accolades given to a tiny number of followers who can be held up as an example. The cult will use converts to bring in more people to bolster the numbers. All the while the congregation is kept busy buying diet books, recipes and health snacks and in turn the industry gets richer. Willingly the congregation hands over their cash and gets nothing in return but promises. They are told to be patient because despite a lifetime of waiting and working and dedication salvation is always just around the corner. Anyone who questions their methods is soon ostracized from the group and silenced. In fact they will have convinced you to silence yourself because to question them only highlights your lack of willpower.

Suppose there was a way out? Suppose there was an alternative? No one is to blame for not questioning their methods. It seems so convincing and there is no alternative on offer, until now that is. I would like to get over the wall and talk to the diet community and see if any are willing to try. Imagine if I could get into the compound to talk to the followers. Whilst their leaders are out of the room I could stand up and make one desperate bid to rescue as many as I could.

ESCAPING THE DIET CULT

"Ladies and gentlemen I don't have much time. I have come from the outside and I can take some of you with me. What you have been told is not true. You can leave here with me tonight. You can live your life without being on a diet ever again"

"That's a lie, he is here to trick us" someone shouts

"No, don't you see. Ask yourselves how long have you been here? How many have lost weight and how many have gained weight?"

A man steps forward "I have been here 20 years and gained weight but that is my doing. I have no self-control. If I stay I can get to my weight I have seen others do it"

"There is no ideal weight" I scream "Its all a lie. Some people do it but very few because they have something different. Its not because of the diet"

A woman steps up "Maybe your right but what do they have? The super slimmers have told us it's the diet that helped them. If we come with you we will get fat"

"Look I don't have much time. The diet was just the vehicle; even they may not know that yet. Trust me once we are outside the compound I can give you similar tools to help you. I am not saying its easy but it can be done.

"I am going" A man shouts

"Don't trust him, stay here. Its safe"

A group of us assemble and we prepare to leave whilst the rest start to look very uncomfortable and plead with the others not to go with me. "Stay here, you know you can't do it. You have failed before. How will you get on without your diet?"

I gather a small group together.

"OK, listen everyone this is not easy and it can be quite a journey with some unexpected consequences. Once we are out of here I can help you but there will be none of the things your used to. No excuses or calorie counting, we may even forget about weight for some time. There are lots of obstacles and no quick fixes or starvation diets, just you. There will be people who try to tell you it won't work but it can. The likelihood is we will not all get through. You have nothing to lose because staying here will make you bigger but the rewards of getting out are tremendous. Are you still with me"

And with that we set off towards the boundary and that day is the very last day of diets and as a group and as individuals we change right there and then. No more calorie counting, diet books recipes or pills. It sounds crazy but it's not. Never having to obsess or even think about food other than when you are hungry. We are the first but many others will follow us once they see it can be done. I am not saying it's easy, but can it really be harder than being told all your life you are a failure and it's your fault. Escaping the cult has to be worth a try. It's natural to be apprehensive but stay close, open your mind and get ready. Come with me, what have you got to lose?

THE JOURNEY HOME

Being over the fence and away from everything you have depended on is concerning. "Now what?" you may say.

Now we are free we have an exciting journey ahead of us and lots to explore. We will be discovering how every achievement from climbing Everest to writing this book starts and finishes in the mind. You will find out that your weight problem is not entirely your fault because the way you are tackling it is making it worse and deeper, binding you tighter into the cult. We will discover along the way how studies have shown that trying to avoid thinking about something is not only impossible but can lead to obsession with the very thing you don't want to think of. That could be worries, food, cigarettes or booze. Ever tried to get something out of your mind and sleep whilst staying awake all night thinking about it? Diets and weight are just the same and become obsessions with calories, weight and food. The very things you don't want. We are going to explore the common reason why almost every supper slimmer and weightless person achieved what they did. How without knowing, they were able to move their thought process to a different level and you will too. Once you do this and use the tools in this book to create a clear concrete future then the obstacles fade into the background. We will examine your Me-n-a which is a kind of mental DNA or autopilot system. By learning how to change the settings and coordinates then you can relax in the knowledge that you are going the right way. Like a satellite navigation system it will take you places you may never have been before as you head for your destination. We have successful interventions and studies that have helped millions of people overcome depression, drug abuse, crime and family problems. Using these tried and tested methods I am going to present you with a series of the best exercises available. You will be able to try them and see which work for you. All this will happen in a new place for many of us. A place where the diet and everything associated with it is gone forever. Here's the scariest bit of all. If you don't think you have any dependence on diets then how does it feel to discard it all. How does it feel to stop the sessions, the coloured food, the pills and starvation regimes? Yes its scary but this journey is exciting and if we make it life will change forever. Its got to be worth a try. All you have to do is decide that its today, right now. You can jump back over the wall to safety or come with us.

"The problems of today can only be solved at a higher level of thinking than that which created them" – **Albert Einstein**

LEVELS OF CHANGE

A leading thinker and developer in the field of Neuro Linguistic Programming, Robert Dilts produced what he called the logical levels of change. Based on earlier work by the anthropologist Gregory Bateson they provide a blueprint for initiating change in individuals. I would argue that the same applies to businesses, football teams or any organisational structure. Although the theory has its critics there is no denying that it provides a useful metaphor when trying to instigate change at various levels. I only discovered this theory recently and yet it seemed to fit almost everything I have done in talk therapy over the years. In my experience I have found this theory fits almost without exception. So much so that its crucial in understanding one of the reasons why diets do not work effectively.

Before we can understand the principals involved we need to gain an understanding of the levels and the order they stack up. Because once you have an idea of how Dilts theory works then you will have an idea why most diets don't and more importantly why 12 Fat Ladies will.

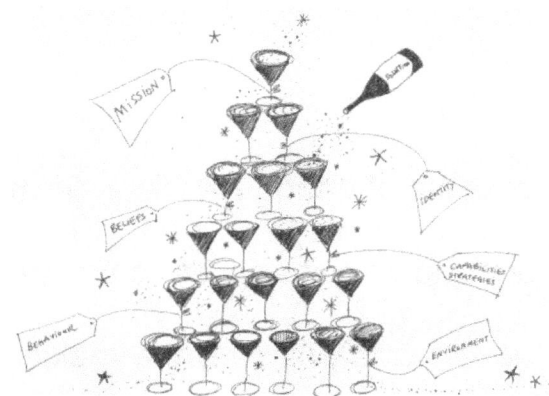

Imagine a champagne fountain with six levels and each level represents an area of behaviour. Then imagine that you were to place your problem at a particular level on the fountain. If we pour champagne in at the top level then it will fill the glass and cascade downwards and so on until it reaches the bottom and all the glasses are full. However if we pour into one of the glasses on level four then it will only fill a certain number of glasses on the way down and it will fill none whatsoever in the levels above. It's the same with change argued Dilts. Should each level represent the place where the problem resides then acting below that will have little lasting effect. In a similar way Dilts argued that a change at a higher level was likely to have an effect on the lower levels but not on the higher. Of course in behavioural terms the idea of having no affect whatsoever on the higher levels does not strictly hold true.

If we use this analogy for behavioural change then it helps to explain why some of the methods we use to instigate long-term change have little or no long-term effect. As a rule we have a tendency to try and change at the wrong level and as such fall back or fail in our attempts to resolve our problem. Following this logic it would be necessary to determine on which level the problem resides and act at the same or any level above. By working on any level above it we have a better chance of lasting change taking place.

In order to explain this in more detail lets look at his levels of change working from the bottom upwards. So to make sense of the theory and how it applies to weight loss and fitness lets carry the solution through the levels and examine the trickle-down effect.

DILTS – LOGICAL LEVELS OF CHANGE

A problem will reside somewhere along the scale and as such can only effectively be resolved at the same or higher level.

- Spirituality/Mission

- Identity

- Beliefs/Values

- Capabilities/Strategies

- Behaviour

- Environment

To gain a greater understanding it is useful to look at each level in more detail.

LEVEL ONE: ENVIRONMENT

This is the very base level of the fountain or pyramid. The environment will be taken to mean the physical place or surroundings where you and your problem reside. This can be taken in the global sense i.e. the country you live in or the place you work or in more immediate terms such as where you are now. This may be your house, car or office. Changes in your environment can often be seen as the answer to any given problem and in one or two cases this may be so. Having said that how common is it for people to make these huge environmental changes in their lives only to find things just feel the same. I knew a very close friend who did just that by emigrating to Australia. Within two years I happened to bump into her in the street and was shocked to even see her in the U.K. I enquired if she was here visiting friends and it transpired not. She confided in me that she had gone there only to find life was really no different. She still had to get up and go to work and pay taxes and do the washing up. Not that there are no fruitful and successful emigrations but in this case it seemed that the change of environment was not the real issue it was something higher up the pyramid. Looking harder she may well have discovered the answer lay at another level. At the opposite end of the scale there are the more immediate changes to your environment such as going outside for some fresh air or holding your sales meeting at a luxurious hotel. In the same way these steps can provide relief but often the resolution lies higher up the scale. When we talk about deep-rooted and lasting change then environment is not ineffective but is certainly the least effective.

Example:

Anne is struggling to gain control of her weight and so decides that some changes to the environment will help. She sets about removing certain foods from the larder and fridge and puts it all in the bin. She also has a number of social functions she thinks are best avoided so as not to put temptation in her way. She may even "Go" to the gym more often as many of us have before but with little heart. It pure mechanics and deep down she may not be sure and would rather be elsewhere. At this level (ENVIRONMENT) there will certainly be some success at least for today. These environmental changes will take away her ability to eat the wrong things but not her desire. In fact Anne probably spends more time thinking about these foods than she normally would. It can be argued that we have all attempted to use the environment to rid ourselves of problems in the short term. According to Dilt's theory this is the bottom of the champagne fountain and there is nowhere for the effects to trickle down to. Will any of these changes trickle up? Does it help you to stop feeling overweight or a failure or even take your mind off the very thing you don't want to think about? You can be the best judge of that but if you have ever dragged yourself down to a gym or out for a walk you will understand that deeper meaning just isn't there.

LEVEL TWO: BEHAVIOUR

Level two is what we physically do as opposed to where we are at any given time. At this level there are global elements and more immediate ones too. Behavioural changes take the form of new production methods or team tactics. This is the level at which you may attempt to do things differently. The problem is approached by changing what you do in any given circumstance and as such changing the short-term result. Once again these changes can be global or local. A business that instructs or trains its unmotivated staff to answer the phones in a different way is making changes to behaviour. They can also be encouraged or ordered to take shorter tea breaks so that production can be increased. None of this will have very much effect on the higher levels because it is unnatural. A football team who have no belief can have the best manager and tactics in the world and still consistently lose games. This is the level where most diets and fitness programmes work but can it filter upwards? Maybe if sustained long enough to become habitual but this is seldom the case. The reason is you are making a behavioural change that is not congruent with your ME-NA Your Mental DNA, It just aint you. What about the trickle-down effect? Surely in most cases the behavioural changes will effect where you are at any given time even if you just FORCE yourself to go to the gym. On the positive there will be many instances where the problem is at this level and so is the solution. Logistical issues can be resolved with behaviour. Once a checking in system is put in place to resolve the problem of returned goods getting lost, bingo!

Example:

Lets go back to Anne again as she attempts to resolve her weight problem with a behavioural change by starting a new diet. Most diets at least in part work at the behavioural level because they are a blueprint or set of instructions on how to eat and exercise. They make no allowance whatsoever for the individuals energy levels or calorific requirements. They demand absolute discipline within preset boundaries. (BEHAVIOUR) If you follow the diet instructions then you will lose weight. The problem seems to be that very few people do keep off the weight they manage to lose. Even though the basic equations less calories and more exercise means weight loss and health. So your changes in behaviour will possibly mean you do not shop or hang out at the same places (ENVIRONMENT). By acting at this level as many do then Anne will achieve a certain amount of success and certainly more than at level one. This strategy will seldom have an effect on any of the above levels. The question is still at which level does the problem reside? Hang on in we are getting to that.

LEVEL THREE: CAPABILITIES/STRATAGIES

In simple terms this is knowledge. The things we all know about any given subject will help us to solve problems better. This can be the training level of your employees or the amount of information given to them. Our government is also keen to encourage higher education so as to have a deeper pool of academic knowledge in the workforce. This level also includes strategies which is how that knowledge is applied and what plans are in place. The government are also keen that the nation is fitter and healthier and so acts at this level by educating its population. We are bombarded with nutritional information on food packaging and the doctors surgery is awash with 5 a day leaflets etc. They are correct in thinking that a better-informed public can make better decisions about its health. An individual at work may also be very knowledgeable about the company strategy and products but will this affect his motivation at a higher level? So to a certain extent you may include diet books, health education and nutrition advice as all adding to our capabilities and strategies.

Example:

Anne decides to do a course on nutrition and exercise or maybe just gets herself the right fitness magazines. Her working knowledge increases and she also reads more about interesting strategies that have worked for others. Slowly she stops counting calories and weighing herself in a diary. She knows what she should and should not eat but that doesn't mean there are good and bad foods. If she does eat any so called bad foods she just ignores it and carries on. (CAPABILITIES).

As she does so then she will be able to avoid certain foods and exercise better and more naturally. (BEHAVIOUR) As a result it feels good to Anne to exercise regularly. (ENVIRONMENT) Theres a feeling now that we are starting to get somewhere. Anne is better informed and is acting upon that information which in turn effects the lower levels.

LEVEL FOUR: BELIEFS/VALUES

These are the deep-rooted beliefs you hold about yourself and those around you. Generalisations built up over time based on life's experience. They become self-replicating as you seek out more and more evidence to prove that your beliefs and values are right. This is where you might here broad statements like. "I am no good with numbers" "I have no willpower" "I am a great people person" "I will never be one of those fit guys you see". Whatever your beliefs or values are you will constantly confirm them time and time again filtering out any evidence to the contrary. The most damaging of these can be negative statements about yourself. These beliefs and values are built up through your life and can be damaging. It's also possible to change your beliefs into more positive ones. It can be a long process but again it becomes easier once you realise what you say and believe about yourself that is unfounded. More importantly here is the incredible power at this level. That's one of the things that 12 Fat Ladies is about.

"If you think you can do a thing or think you can't do a thing, you're right."

Henry Ford

Example:

"I have always been overweight its just the way I am, it runs in the family". Perhaps if that belief was to change and from today you had a different belief about yourself. "That's all behind me now, I am determined to change things for the better and what's more I can". During our sessions we help you to do that and now you really have some power. You are really in control because your goal is crystal clear in your mind. You have set your brain on autopilot and it has set a course. Like being on a cruise ship you have no real need to worry about arriving because it's inevitable. Instead you can relax and enjoy the journey. Because of this new mindset you have no real need to think about food all day every day because the small changes you make naturally will guide you to your destination. (BELIEFS) On that journey you will be interested in health and start to read health magazines instead of diet magazines. As your knowledge increases you find it easier to eat foods that give you more energy and vitality. (CAPABILITIES) Of course your behaviour will change as time goes by. If you are set on a course why would you divert from that by not staying active or eating junk? (BEHAVIOUR) As time progresses you will find you have less time for TV and more time for leisurely pursuits. (ENVIRONMENT) Now Anne is really feeling the benefits and has little doubt in her mind as she resets her ME-NA and only has her goal in mind. Her deep rooted belief frees here from the diet regime and she settles into a slightly different lifestyle.

LEVEL FIVE: IDENTITY/MISSION

This is who you really are and the role you play in various situations. Are you the dogsbody or the head of the household? The life and soul of the party or the wallflower? Most of all are you a fitness geek or a couch potato? We all have an identity as a person and that shifts depending on the role we are playing and who with. If you met a friend in the street and she was with a stranger how would she describe you after you walked away. "Oh that john, he is such a funny guy" "I used to work with him he was really good at his job". "That's Irene she goes to the same gym as me, I wish I had her dedication"

Your identity is malleable and can be changed with time but you cannot hide from yourself. I have worked with people who want to become non-smokers and a crucial time for them is the normalising phase. The time when they are non smokers and friends have stopped asking "Still not smoking then?" The normalising stage where the new behaviours have no novelty value or kudos because its just you. Remember the first weeks of the job you do now and all the insecurities you had? As you grow in your profession it becomes part of your identity and mission. In my terms it normalises and then you can continue to grow by study and experience to be at the top of your profession. In the marvellous book "Mind Hacks" by Tom Stafford and Matt Webb there is a similar theory which talks about how we follow a cycle. At the top is the phase of normality in which you do all the day to day tasks your used to such as washing up and going to work etc. Then theres the dreaming phase where you wander what it would be like to do all those things in a new country with a warmer climate and more spare time. Many people would stop there but other might move on to experimentation and get some flights or check out careers in their chosen country. Following this there is the experimentation phase where they move abroad and adapt to the new way of life. Finally they return to the top of the cycle as all these things become normal in their life once more. Applying this same theory to health and fitness we find many people get beyond dreaming and as far as experimenting. If through mental training you could normalise these traits can you see how powerful this level can be. Its here that health and fitness becomes part of your mental DNA or ME-N-A as I call it.

Example:

You become the amateur fitness guru in your household. Friends say to you "Can you recommend some good food supplements or a good workout to set me off" "Hey you keep fit don't you? I need some help". This is your identity and that's why people come to you for help. (IDENTITY) This confirms your beliefs that you deserve that reputation and so your beliefs are embedded (BELIEFS) Your knowledge is quite extensive as it would be for anyone who has a keen interest in their own health and wellbeing. (CAPABILITIES) By now it goes without saying that you would enjoy a healthy diet and a healthy relationship with food. You are not afraid of any foods in particular and there are no bad foods or foods to avoid. It's simply a case of moderation and enjoying everything you eat. (BEHAVIOUR) You may well enjoy a night in front of the telly on occasions but get a little agitated when a day or two goes by without doing something active. You have a real need to get to the gym, have a run or go for a walk. (ENVIRONMENT)

LEVEL SIX: SPIRITUALITY/MISSION

This is big time top-level stuff and determines your real mission in life. Anything from Mother Teresa to just being the mother of the household. It the purpose in life that is at your very core and this shapes your entire destiny and any changes here will cascade down to the very bottom of the pyramid. Some people's spiritual purpose is obvious whilst others is not. A man who dedicates his life to religion or science as well as an entire adult life taken up with the care of an elderly relative or family member are all peoples mission in life. This is the pinnacle and if it's right there's a lovely view from up here. How many times have you heard someones real motivation is their kids, to run with them and live longer. Changes at this level will cascade down like a torrent but to make changes at this level takes a lot of work or sometimes it can happen in an instant. A single incident can and has changed some peoples lives forever. Lord Baden Powell saw how interested and independent young boys became when trained in survival skills. After writing his book Scouting for Boys he is responsible for a movement that boasts 28 million members. In other least recognisable ways the unselfish acts of family members who are dedicated to the care of their own. Animal and human rights activists who lose their own freedom to fight for what they believe is true and right. We all have this sense of Mission and belief and it does not have to be so grand as some of these examples. However, if and when changes are made at this level they cascade down from the very peak of our existence. In his amazing book "Man's Search For Meaning" Victor Frankle talks of his life in the Nazi death camps and how he used his time to study humankind and the attributes of those that survived. He knew that his purpose was to survive and tell this story to the world and he did. Even in these circumstances he found a purpose that he believes kept him alive. Our changes do not have to be so grand but can be more personal. When they happen at this level they hold a real power to change everything forever. How similar this is to the stories at the beginning of the book of super slimmers and how the effect on their loved ones was a turning point bringing them the crunch.

Example:

I am sure this is a very common story you will have heard many times. A person who is overweight and not very active is constantly bullied and called names at school. It affects their self-confidence and is carried through into adult life. One day a person they don't even know makes a remark about their weight. Something changes on that day and they decide enough is enough. They have reached the CRUNCH and it acts as a central point to shift everything in their lives forever. They become devoted to their health and helping others do the same. They are completely focused on their desired outcome and can clearly see the end result of their efforts. (SPIRITUALITY/MISSION) In doing so they are now the health guru in the family, community or country. His self-confidence grows every day as people congratulate him on his success. (IDENTITY) His knowledge is increased as he becomes more and more interested in the workings of the human body and mind. (CAPABILITIES) He has a different view of health, wellbeing and exercise and so is more inclined to choose the right foods and enjoy exercise and sports. (BEHAVIOUR) It goes without saying that his immediate environment will change in numerous ways from how he spends his leisure time to where he works. (ENVIRONMENT)

When change takes place at the highest level then we see the power of humankind. Mahatma Ghandi, Mother Teresa and Martin Luther King, people who changed the lives of millions forever because of it. Lots of people lived in similar environments or had better skills and shared their beliefs. The striking thing about these particular individuals was that they held a deep spiritual belief in why they were here.

DILTS & ME?

Once we choose to accept this way of thinking then its interesting to try building in an issue of our own. This does not just apply to health and fitness but to any personal, company or organisational issue. By examining the issue of health and fitness we can measure the various interventions and see if we can agree on which level they apply. Once we are in agreement on which level the problem resides we should be able to see how we can have the greater effect.

On the next page is a brief summary and explanation of Dilts theory.

Level	Questions/Answers	For Example
Spirituality/Purpose	Your spiritual purpose in life. Your ethics and long term goals	"Why am I here" "What is my purpose in life"
Identity/Mission	Who you think you are. The labels we give ourselves. Identities or roles will change depending on the situation	"Am I the head of the household or the dogsbody?" "The ideas guy or the minute taker"
Beliefs/Values	Often unfounded beliefs built up over time from experience and influence. You will develop an ability to confirm these to yourself over time regardless	"You can't trust men" "Traffic wardens are bad" "You can't teach an old dog new tricks"
Capabilites/Stratagies	The skills and resources you have available to you. Either academic, physical or mental abilities	"I am good at my job" "I have experienced this before"
Behaviour	What you will actually do or say in any given situation	"I am starting a diet" "I study every Sunday evening"
Environment	The place you are at any given time, like all the others this can change dependant on the situation	"This place gets me down" "I love being here" Living in a poor country, being at work or home for Christmas are all different environments

You are free to make your own assessment in all these cases but I am going to place my problem of health and fitness at the level of beliefs/values. This is the lowest level I can possibly put it considering I am not forced to overeat by my environment although it could help. In the same way behaviour is a factor in maintaining my on-going problem it is still rooted at a higher level than that. As for capabilities I would personally be lying if I said I just had no idea that what I was eating would make me put on weight in relation to my activity. Both behaviour and environment are easy enough to change if they were the real core causes. So the highest credible level I can put this issue is Beliefs/Values.

Level	Explanation	Problem level	Solution A	Solution B	Solution C	Solution D	Solution E
6	Spirituality						
5	Identity						
4	Beliefs/Values						
3	Capabilities						
2	Behaviour						
1	Environment						

According to the theory it is necessary to act at a level at or above your problem to have a real and lasting effect. So now we can place each of our proposed solutions into the chart to see which level they act upon.

1 Government Advice

This will be things like the 5 a day campaign or other information campaigns whether through leaflets in a doctors surgery, working with women or youth groups. Warnings about foods with high fat content and advice on how much bacon or beef to eat etc.

Level: Capabilities

2 Food Labeling

This will take the form of various standards of colour coding and labeling to advise on fat content as well as nutritional breakdown and contents of any given food. These programmes tend to be voluntary as manufacturers buy into the health market.

Level: Capabilities

3 Physical Intervention

Considered by some to be the extreme where surgery or physical intervention is involved. This could include gastric bands or jaw wiring. There are also forms of liposuction and surgery that will physically remove excess fat from the body.

Level: Behaviour

4 Diets

These take many forms but broadly speaking you can expect a set of "rules" to adhere to where food intake is concerned. They can be policed in numerous ways even to the point where your food is delivered and you have no influence over its content. The general aim of the diet will be to deprive you of calories and as such reduce your weight.

Level: Behaviour

5 12 Fat Ladies

The absolute "Anti-diet" which in effect has no nutritional rules or advice whatsoever. It allows you to take control and responsibility back from the industry. In its place it provides a series of tried and tested techniques which are harmless yet powerful. It allows you to use your own mind in the same way as every other person who has achieved anything has always done. From giving up drugs to climbing Everest, from marathon runners to super slimmer's.

Level: Identity

The levels above can be argued and you are welcome to switch them around as you see fit, however I can clearly see a very strong case for Psychological intervention rather than physical. The final test is to look once more at the chart and pick out which intervention is about physical action or control and which are about using mental control.

With this knowledge its now worth taking a look at the super slimmers in more detail and discovering not just the pattern of behaviour but at which level it operates.

I LOST 3 STONE IN A WEEK *RESULTS NOT TYPICAL*

Laura Powell is a 27 year old attractive, healthy and presumably happy young woman by all accounts considering her upcoming dream wedding. Like most brides she will relish celebrating her wedding with loved ones and being the centre of attention on her special day. After years of planning, the day arrives and Laura prepares to fit snuggly into her size 12/14 wedding dress. She is also very proud and has every right to be because she was the winner of the Rosemary Connelly Bridal slimmer of the year. She is a size 12/14 average size but until relatively recently she weighed 23 stone and was a size 26. Thanks to Rosemary Connelly something changed in her life and so after enrolling in the class she couldn't be happier. Like many of her devotees Rosemary interviewed Laura in her private studio to ask how it felt to win the award. In the video which is one of many she tells of how great it feels to be healthy, have more energy and feel gorgeous on her wedding day and indeed she did. Then rosemary asks the key question "At what point did you decide to lose weight?" Laura relates a familiar story. She was concerned about a new job which would involve flying and this may become a problem due to her size. Around about the same time she was engaging in one of her favourite pastimes less and less. Theme parks. She always loved theme park rides and on this particular day she had headed down to the theme park and got on her first ride. What transpired then was an embarrassing situation in which two members of staff were required to fit her into the seat. At that point Laura said "I can't do this" and walked away. Whilst at home she was able to think about what had happened. She was also keen to marry and have children at that time whilst seeing people who were what she says Size 12 and 14 being asked to have obesity checks prior to pregnancy. "I thought if that's happening to them then what about me?" She says "It was kind of an accumulation of everything really and so that's when I joined Rosemary Connelly"

A fantastic achievement and brilliant PR for Rosemary who has numerous award winners on her own web TV channel. These stories are inspirational and most likely encourage others to think "If only I could do that" If only I had the determination to succeed then.. but I cant. Why do I fail and succeed, fail and succeed? How determined had she been or was she just lucky?

Wayne tells a similar story to a newspaper. Like many loving parents he had been walking his daughter home from school one day when he noticed she was visibly upset. He pressed her to tell him what was wrong and eventually she did.

With tears in her eyes she said "It was obesity day today at school" and the teacher had said "Obese people die earlier than healthy people" She was very concerned her dad would not be around much longer. He had been in an accident at work some years ago which reduced his mobility and his weight had ballooned.

Wayne said "It really hit home what my weight had done to me and my family" He had not realized how depressed his weight had made him, always having to buy the biggest size, thinking people were sniggering at him behind his back "Now" he said "It was effecting the rest of my family and I had to do something about it"

That was when Wayne joined "Slimming World" He has lost more than 7 stones and never looked back. "I am alive once more, loving life with my family and making up for lost time. Slimming World has made an amazing difference in all our lives in one way or another"

Another inspiring story this time some great PR from Slimmers World.

Emmerdale and comedy actress Pauline Quirke reports her story when at 20 stone she had to ask for a seat belt extension on an aircraft "I felt like crap to do that in front of my husband and kids" she said. "I was clinically obese" She explains that means "it's a threat to your life" Shortly afterwards she started the Lighter Life plan and has lost eight stone.

This time it's the Lighter Life plan? The stories fill our Sunday papers and slimming websites and are an inspiration to others to do the same. But that's just it, we don't do the same do we? They are portrayed as special and are more hard working and dedicated than us and it feels awful and it feels like our fault. There are endless stories of how people of all ages and sizes had used one diet or another having an incredible impact on their weight. These are the kind of stories that are used to convince us that diets work. They are held up as examples of what you could do if you had the courage and determination this time to see it through. Notwithstanding that every one of them has certainly worked hard and deserves credit for manufacturing a turnaround in lifestyle that is mind boggling. The stories are similar and inspiring in many ways but interestingly the diet plan used, the vehicle to weight loss is different in each case and there are hundreds more they could have chosen. In fact there are as many stories as there are weight loss schemes. Bridie Coulter the Connelly 40+ slimmer of the year 2010 had reached size 44 and had to have disability rails fitted in the house until her doctor told her she may not be around in another 12 months unless she did something. That day she decided to change her life.

Kerry Pillai is now a super fit slimmer training for a marathon and to be a fitness instructor. She has a new life and feels like a new person after realizing that her weight might stop her having children. The 30-year-old dropped from 19st 8lb to 9st 2lb after she was told she could not have the fertility treatment she needed to conceive until she lost her excess weight.

"I realised I'd wasted an entire decade not doing anything," she said. "When my husband wanted to go out I said I was ill or too tired.

"But after visiting the fertility clinic I set a goal to turn my life around by 30.

"In the last year I've done everything I always wanted to."

All of these stories are common and whilst people like this are rightly proud of their achievements and hard work they are paraded by the diet companies as the norm. They are held up as beacons to what you could do with the same dedicated hard work. But when you start to dig a little deeper you see a pattern emerging that can often go unnoticed. They all reached what I call the "crunch" The point at which everything in the brain shifts around just enough to switch their focus of attention in a slightly different direction.

These stories are often remarkably similar and that's not surprising. Children or them being bullied or upset, the potential to never realize their dream or the embarrassing situation that although often minor it seems to flick a switch and its crunch time. Once you have had the crunch then the focus has changed and in reality there is no need for diet plans or calorie counting or dragging yourself off to the gym. They work as a vehicle I agree but your focus is now on the goal. You can clearly see the end result and your objective will be achieved without the bind of micro managing your life. Your brain has switched and you know it. At this stage you are charging towards your imagined future throwing every obstacle out of the way. Pretty soon normality sets in and that's just what you do, it becomes a way of life. The achievement is set in stone for you now and it was always going to be that way. In a similar way to an ex-smoker you no longer consider good foods or bad foods like a smoker hardly ever thinks about not smoking. The things you craved exist in a different mental compartment and are easier to either avoid or abstain all together. You no longer have to think too much about not eating them, why would you? They are bad. Where you used to drag yourself off to the gym or make excuses you now feel edgy if you have not been for a few days.

What I am arguing is that once you hit the crunch in your life then your brain and subconscious take over. You are on autopilot towards your destination. Once you reach this stage then obstacles fade into the background and the only focus is the goal. Concern and anguish about small disasters become irrelevant because whenever something trys to blow you off course you reset the focus and carry on. How does this help you? You can't just create some kind of traumatic episode to boost your weight loss programme. That's true but I will argue that through years of working with self-destructive behaviour using numerous tried and tested therapies I can help you make some mental adjustments at the right level. Once that happens then in the same way as the super slimmers everything else will follow suit.

12 Fat Ladies ™ is the building of an idea that is working right now for millions of people with self-destructive behaviours whilst the diet industry has got everyone else looking in the wrong direction. I am going to explain how the different motivations of the people we described earlier in this chapter are what really count. The key is the inner belief system that influences every decision you make and your mental autopilot which sets the target and moves relentlessly forward. In most cases its an invisible influence that hides behind every decision and

everything we are willing to accept for ourselves.   Knowing it is there is the first step to questioning where it gets these blueprints from and why they should be adjusted. But first we need a metaphor to grasp how this secret record keeper gets its information and often keeps false records about you and acts as if they were true.

ME-N-A?

It was 1951 when two scientists, James Watson and Francis Crick started work to discover the structure of DNA (Deoxyribonucleic Acid). In 1953 they published their structure which showed the now common form of double helix and received the Nobel Prize in 1962. Since those early days we have come a long way and even young school children will recognize the DNA helix as the blue print for our physical characteristics. It consists of a tiny coil up to a meter in length over a single DNA molecule. It is divided into sections known as genes and provides a code that we inherit from our parents. One half from our father and the other from our mother just as each of them did a generation before. This unique code determines our physical characteristics as each gene is responsible for a particular task. The DNA determines everything about us from hair colour, eye colour and even a tendency towards particular diseases etc. This blueprint provides the instruction manual for every individual human being and is unique to them alone. This code has been passed on and changed through generation after generation only to end with you as an individual. You are so individual that the U.K. now holds a DNA database which includes 5.2% of its population for crime detection purposes. Your DNA will have a profound effect on your life as it determines how you are made but we all know that this is not the end of the story. Just because you may have a tendency towards a particular disease there is no guarantee you will live long enough to die from it because of outside factors. You may not even live to pass this tendency on at all to your offspring. In a way the DNA is purely the building blocks of the physical human being. What you choose to do with that human being is entirely up to you and is subject to change.

The concept of DNA is now universal in our society and we have no problem understanding how it works. This being the case it should be quite easy to grasp the concept of something I call "ME-N-A".

THE ROBOT

I have a little robot that goes around with me

I tell it what I'm thinking; I tell it what I see

I tell my little robot all my hopes and fears

It listens and remembers everything it hears

At first my little robot followed my commands

But after years of training it's gotten out of hand

It doesn't care what's right or wrong

or what is false or true

No matter what I try now, it tells ME what to do.

By Anon

ME-N-A (MENTAL DNA) © DAWSON 1999

There was still a slight chill to the early summer breeze as the Texas sun rose through the trees. Jethro stumbles up the rocky unkept path pushing overhanging branches to one side with his one free arm. Under the other he cradles a small baby piglet. Behind him follows his excited new bride anticipating the sight of what is to be her marital home for the first time. Jethro stumbles against the steep craggy rock and his foothold is not helped by his worn grey unlaced boots. His leathery hands grip into the dirty protruding tree roots to his left forcing more dirt into his crumbling fingernails. His pretty young bride wears only slippers and the tattered remains of a dress that has seen much better days. Finally as they reach the top of the hill the house comes into view. Jethro emerges from the woods, squinting into the morning sun as his new bride joins him by his side. He stands proudly with one hand on his hip chewing the blade of grass stuck to his lower lip intently. Brushing her long straggly hair from her face his new wife stands by him to survey the scene before her.

In a clearing there is a broken wooden hut with a hint of smoke cascading from the chimney into the morning sky. The front door is barely on its hinges and the front garden is strewn with rubbish and scrap metal of various kinds. Rats can be seen brazenly scurrying amongst open bin bags and waste food scrap before disappearing back under the front porch. The rotting wooden frames contain a small number of unbroken panes whilst the rest are damaged or missing. Pausing next to her new husband her eyes widen to accommodate the incredible scene before her. She grips a handful of black knotted locks as her hand stops on top of her head and she gasps.

"Well" Says Jethro pulling up his tattered dungarees. "What d'yah think"

"Oh my" She exclaims "I know you said you were rich, but I never dreamed you were this rich"

One of the most defining strategies within the world of talking therapy is that the client is the expert and as such can define their own success. The reason being that success is relative. Success can be walking to the shops or up the stairs or putting on a pair of jeans. Success can be finishing that marathon or hitting that dress size. Its up to the individual to define it from their own perspective. This is one of the reasons the questionnaire featured in this book is worthy of some time and a pen, not just scanning through it. Its vital to begin with the end in mind no matter what that end is for you. Once your goal is concrete then like many of the super slimmers you will power towards success and obstacles will fade into the background.

As the amusing story above illustrates, its what you perceive as success that really counts.

Like many of you I find myself frequenting city centre shopping areas where you will often come across people selling the Big Issue magazine. If you are not aware of the Big Issue then look it up. They are a business designed to provide honest work for homeless people by selling an excellent quality magazine to the public for a small commission. In this way they are able to support themselves and get a foothold back into mainstream society. A brilliant and yet simple idea. Having met and worked with some of these characters I am aware that they are often articulate and intelligent people who have come across difficult circumstances. On some occasions they have not coped well and as such need strategies to survive. Crime as well as drugs and alcohol are common problems causing their lives to crash down around them. Whilst selling on the streets it is noticeable that some develop their own individual sales strategy through experience. One man in particular struck me so much that I bought a coffee at the shop across the road and observed him. He was a jovial character and seemed to actually love what he was doing. Yes he loved this job and loved his customers or so it seemed. As I sipped my coffee hoping he would not notice me it became apparent that his love for his job and his customers may or may not be genuine. After all he was homeless and probably forced to do this job as a last resort. This was irrelevant to me, to him and most importantly to his customers. What was important to us all was the perception that he loved the job, not just loved the job but actually selling the magazine was secondary. As a result he sold noticeably more magazines than anyone. After sitting there for a while it was clear he had built up a regular client group who enjoyed their short engagement with this character. I could not hear the words but I could see the smiles on the faces of people as they walked away whether they had a Big Issue in their hands or not.

In the car on the way home I was considering the talents that I had been witnessing. It dawned on me that regardless of what the guy selling the Big Issue did he would achieve good sales using the talent he had. No doubt he was happy to do that but could he have done better?

Lets say we take this same guy and put him in any sales environment such as timeshare or even health club membership etc. He has a great talent for working with people and being able to approach strangers without giving offence. He would no doubt be great at that particular job and would be able to make a better living for himself. The point is he has no aspirations to do so and as such is happy with the achievement he attains on a day-to-day basis. There is no particular problem with anyone being happy with any level of attainment but the question remained, could he do better? It's at this point I started to develop the idea of a mental DNA. It's not in our genes or make up but is built in to our brains through consistent conditioning. It tells us where our comfort zone is and determines what we are willing to accept in our lives on a day-to-day basis. It draws an exact parallel with the real DNA in many ways. I was reading an inspiring book recently by the entrepreneur Duncan Ballatyne in which he says "Drop me off in a town anywhere in the world with nothing and in no time at all I will find a way to make money". I am sure he would not be offended if I was to suggest he is not the smartest or most talented guy in the world. Neither am I and neither are you so what makes him think he can say that? Perhaps his mental DNA or what I call his ME-NA is different.

The author and self-help guru Anthony Robbins tells about when he was out walking late one night when a drunk approaches him and says

"Can you spare a dime?"

Anthony pulls out his money clip and says "Is that all you want?"

The guys says "Yeh"

Anthony then gives him some words of wisdom "Life will give you whatever you ask of it" and he hands him the dime.

The guy then looks Anthony in the eye and says "You are weird man" and staggers off.

The interesting part of the story is that as Anthony went back to his room he was asking himself "What's different between me and that guy?" Well maybe I have an answer, maybe it is the ME-N-A

These two cases are extremes and yet we all have a ME-NA that tells us what we are and what we accept in our lives as well as what we are capable of. What sort of car do you drive if any and why? Do you even own a car? What sort of job do you do now and how much better are you at it than your boss and even his boss? Don't we all get what our mental DNA tells us we are entitled to? The mental DNA I am talking about is like a barometer for what you will accept in your life, relationships and finances.

Our physical DNA is fixed when we are born and therefore we are forced to work with the physical characteristics we are born with. If you are tall you're tall and that's it. The difference with ME-NA is that it is constantly changing and therefore you are not stuck with the same options and self-beliefs. It's pretty tough to change it don't get me wrong but it does change over time either by your physical intervention or just naturally. Let's say we go back to our homeless guy and we get over a few hurdles. We would need to get him through an interview or convince an employer he was worth a shot. Just doing these things would help him realize the immense talent he has which exceeds some people who have been in the job for years. So he overcomes the hurdle and finds himself smartly dressed and enrolling more people into his gym membership scheme than anyone else. For years he is a star performer doing exactly what he does right now. Engaging with members of the public in a warm friendly way through his huge personality. The expectations from his lifestyle and income would change over time and normalise. This is the new ME-NA which tells him where he now is in his life.

So tomorrow yet again he finds himself back on the streets selling the Big Issue. What then? He no longer belongs in this world but if he stays long enough he soon will. The very first thing on his mind will be to get back to where he feels right. At this point he has to act fast before he normalizes this existence. This would never happen but it does indicate how two people of similar talents can find themselves in very different places. Not only in different places but quite happy to accept them. There are many reasons why we develop our own unique ME-N-A and some of them do come from our parents or lack of them although not in a 50:50 proportion as with the DNA. Our culture plays a massive part as well as upbringing and influence from friends and associates. This blueprint for your life and its expectations is as real as DNA. It affects everything you do and every decision you make at any one time. Taking the point of the earlier story the humour was gained from the fact that the lovely young bride was surprisingly happy to accept terrible standards and is happy to do so. Without knowing anything about her we would of course assume she would be devastated at the prospect of her new marital home. In fact she was over the moon at the prospect. The reason the story is funny is because our ME-NA tells us that she was going to live in a place way below our own standards. The sometimes uncomfortable question now is what's your ME-N-A telling you right now? Are you settling for second best or only the best in health, life and relationships? I'll leave that with you and maybe you could put the kettle on and have a cup of tea before we move on.

Lots of people are happy to decide that their lack of fitness or excessive weight gain is in some way related to physical DNA make up and they may be right. How many including yourself are willing to attribute these same things to your ME-N-A? A measure of what you are willing to accept for yourself and how you are willing to feel about that? Our mental DNA is not fixed but is based on our experiences and the messages we give ourselves. Your mental DNA can be trained to demand more from your daily expectations in every aspect of your life. What seems to have passed our fad diet, fast fix, miracle pill society is that our ME-N-A has the power to overcome anything our physical make up can throw at us. Once the ME-N-A changes then everything else has no choice but to fall into line.

OUR OWN ROBOTS

The ME-N-A is a term of reference for our own little robot. He is locked away deep in the mind and sits in a control room but has instant access to the ME-N-A and will refer to it prior to any decision. Here he has a handle on moods, assumptions as well as the information he has collated over the years which makes up our ME-N-A. Depending on the incoming information he will make decisions that affect our reactions to disease, interactions with strangers, achievements and assumptions.

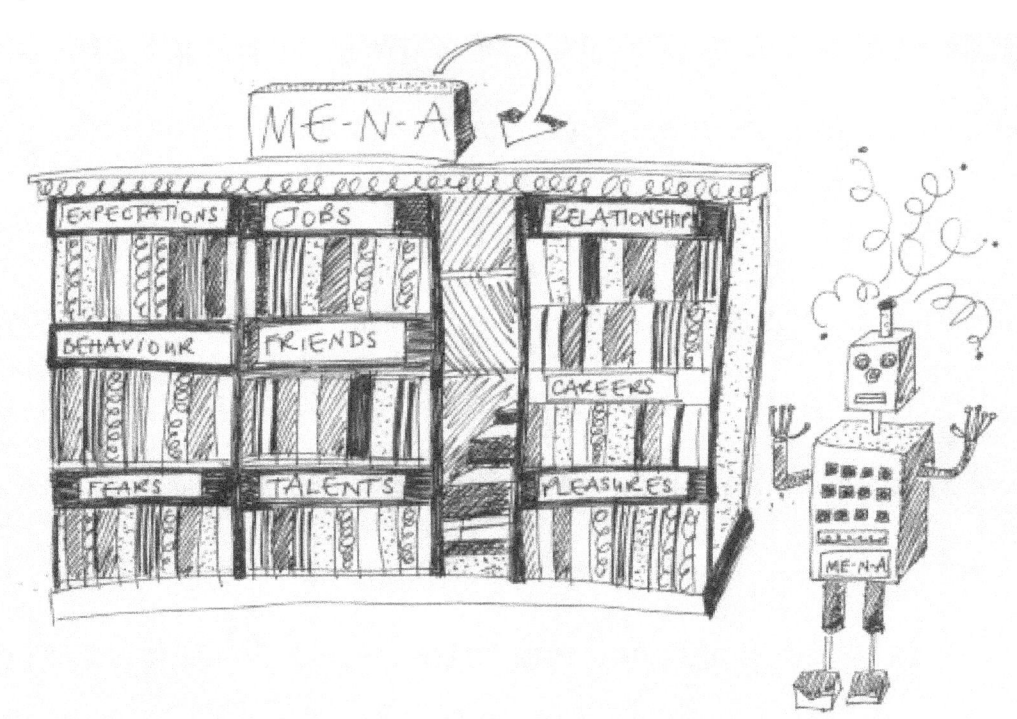

The problem with this robot is he has no real language and so its impossible to speak to him directly. He seems to peek through a small slit in the mind and depending on what he sees will keep adding to his files. He is often unsure of the quality of the information but will use it just the same. He is known to make broad sweeping assumptions about single incidents and file them away. He has no idea what is real or imagined and yet he lends more weight to information that confirms what he knows. One of his particular foibles is that he has no negatives. If you ask him not to think of pink elephants he has to look them up first and so forces you to think of them.

He is the oldest part of the mind and in the early age of mankind was vital for survival. The conscious mind is way too slow in assessing danger and so the subconscious watches, assesses and acts quickly to keep you safe.

In reality there is a lot of evidence that confirms unconscious activity. In one experiment a group of students were asked to sit in a room and watch the hand of a clock rotate. At any time of their own choosing they were asked to simply press a button which switched on a light. All they had to do was note where the hand on the clock was at the instant they made that decision. This would tell the experimenters at which point they had "decided" to press the button. A simple enough process until they were wired up to brainwave detection equipment. This is when something strange happened. The scientists were able to detect significant brain activity prior to the decision. It was as if there was something deep down which was deciding that they were going to decide? If this was the case then the implications are plain. If our decisions are at deeper levels and are based on false information about us then we may have already set ourselves up to fail. Could this be why the higher levels of intervention are so powerful? Is it because they are the levels that control every decision good or bad through reference to the ME-N-A? If that's so then if those reference files are wrong we are going to make poor decisions. What if the files say we are weak willed or bad with numbers or shy in crowds. This will drastically affect our conscious thoughts and actions. A stronger ME-N-A would give different messages about what we eat, who we have as friends and every other fabric of our lives.

If we could find better ways of communicating with the robot then his interpretation of what we want would improve. It becomes apparent that we need to find ways to act at a higher level than the physical one. These are the skills adopted with the therapies contained in this book.

MY VERY OWN OBSESSION

Some time ago I had decided to do some work in my bathroom. Feeling I was quite handy I felt capable of swapping the bathroom suite and plumbing in a new one as well as the related tasks. When plumbing in the bath it was a struggle for space but I popped in the rubber washer and ensured the fitting was as tight as possible. Once the water was switched on, guess what? It leaked. I disconnected it and tried again and every time I tightened it more and had to buy new washers because the ones I had ripped several times. In the end I took the bath out and tightened it so tight there was no way it was going to leek. Yes you have guessed it. In desperation I called a plumber friend who explained what I was doing wrong. The way to seal these fittings was to just tighten with fingers then a quarter turn with pliers. That's all. It transpired that the tighter I fitted the nut the more I was destroying the washer which was designed to make the seal. It worked perfectly and I realised I had been doing the exact opposite of what was required. The less it worked the more I tightened making the problem worse. Studies are starting to show that people with addictive behaviours can act in a similar way. The process seems to work the same way regardless of what the thought is. It can be tobacco, drugs, food or even worries.

"Polivy and Herman (1985) indicated that dieting generally causes subsequent overeating. They cite several converging sources of evidence suggesting that the restraint of eating is a reliable precursor of binge eating and overweight. It seems, then, that the attempt to avoid thoughts of food may lead to a later preoccupation with such thoughts."

Journal personality and social sciences 1987 vol 53 No1.5-13

We attempt to push the thought from our minds but in doing so actually have to think about it. Then we notice we are thinking about it and try harder. Eventually the thought goes away and the slightest thing can make it come back. At this stage it appears that some of the people who were most effective at banishing the thought tend to fall victim to the rebound effect. This is where the smallest indiscretion results in a huge relapse into the addictive behaviour. The studies go even further in suggesting that in real world conditions outside of the laboratory their results could be magnified. Our own experience will surely bear out the laboratory evidence when struggling with addiction of any kind. We struggle not to think about the very thing we want to avoid and then like an avalanche we have not only returned to the behaviour but had that huge satisfying binge along with its accompanying feeling of gratification followed by guilt and failure. There is one great redeeming feature from the laboratory experiments and that is distraction. They claim that an active interest in a single positive distracter was effective against the rebound effect. Our minds can only hold between 7 and 9 thoughts at any one time. It's a bit like being asked to carry thoughts and then another one needs picking up. Your mind can pick it up but has to put another one down. This fact is well known by magicians who use it to great effect to distract your attention during their act. Hypnotists use it to confuse your senses and desensitise you and access your subconscious. What the studies show is that when you want to avoid food the very last thing that is going to help you is trying to avoid thinking about it. In most diet regimes then this is exactly what you are asked to do. These studies suggest that an appropriate distractor is far more likely to help. I am suggesting that when the distractor is at a level of belief and values and when the distractor involves a clear achievable end result in full colour. When you learn how to smell, see, taste and hear your goal. Maybe now you are starting to see how the deeply embedded and emotional decisions made by the super slimmers were so powerful. These emotional incidents became for them a huge distractor magnet drawing them towards their success. All the previous obstacles became grey and faded into the background. The thoughts they once tried desperately to avoid are no longer on their mental radar. That's why some of the exercises in 12 Fat Ladies are to help you develop similar crystal clear goals. There is nothing more powerful in helping you focus and avoid the rebound trap we have all fallen into, some of us to the point of obsession. The report above ends by saying that there is little to be gained by trying not to think of something. The message is that we need to be able to see the end in a crystal clear way involving as many senses and emotions as possible.

PUTTING THE PIECES TOGETHER

From the other side of the fence and a safe distance from the cult things start to look very different. Some of the self-destructive behaviours we indulged in have scientific explanations to support them. More importantly we can start to see the diet industry which we held in such high esteem is a sham. It held us trapped on a rollercoaster of hope and success followed by failure and even despair. Even those who we jokingly call the "weightless" would join the cult if the need ever arose because they believed in it too. The level at which it worked either had no long term effect or made the problem worse. The super slimmers have often been unwitting conspirators in their success. Now we know how we could do the same or better if only we too could reach a point similar to the crunch. We now have an understanding of how the decisions we make on a day to day basis beneath our conscious minds are often based on false beliefs about ourselves. Serious studies have indicated how and why abstinence often results in a huge relapse rather than just a minor setback. Whilst we try to avoid thoughts they return to a point of obsession. The Yo-yo dieting, binge eating and false messages we have given ourselves all make sense now. Armed with this knowledge we can now spot and understand what these behaviours are and know that its not our fault. But more importantly we need to start the fight back. The 12 Fat Ladies are the bullets but before you take aim let me tell you a little about the weapons.

THE WEAPONS OF CHOICE

SOLUTION FOCUSED BRIEF THERAPY

Steve de Shazer and Insoo Kim Berg developed Solution Focused Brief Therapy in America in the 1980s. Noticing that most talking therapies attempted to find the problem and tackle that they decided to start from the solution.

It works around some very clever and basic principles. We would all agree that no one is perfect and as such there can be no one capable of having the perfect problem. In a nutshell there are days when they are just not as good at having the problem. This being the case then surely if we can find the times the client is not very good at having his problem then there lies the solution. These are the times that De Shazer called "exceptions". An examination of these times in more depth will allow the client to find change. The language and ethos of Solution Focused Therapy is about helping to elicit an imagined future without the particular problem and what steps will guide the client to that future. The model is completely non-judgmental and unobtrusive. It supports the clients thought processes and reminds them of their own resources and strengths. Widespread research shows to be effective in 65-83% of cases in an average of 4-5 sessions even for serious problems.

NEURO LINGUISTIC PROGRAMMING

Neuro Linguistic Programming (NLP) has been adopted worldwide as a working tutorial for how the human mind works.

It's described as the operator's manual for the brain and helps individuals understand better how this magnificent tool can work for us and against us. We often say how we are teaching people what they already know but without the formal knowledge the brain can easily control us instead of the other way round. The skills developed in NLP are real and applicable to everyday life. The results of NLP are well documented and if you have come this far you will already be aware of its basic premise. There is no better and fun way to learn about NLP than by practice in a group or workshop. NLP works from a basic set of rules or assumptions and expands upon those into a real command of everyday thoughts and actions that lead to greater success. Search a million websites and read a thousand books, absorb all you can about this brilliant resource

CLINICAL HYPNOSIS

Hypnosis is a naturally occurring psychological process that when used deliberately makes positive use of relaxation, strong concentration and the imagination.

When a person is able to skilfully create concentration, induce relaxation, and stimulate the imagination in oneself and others, the effect can be powerful! It is almost like creating a "virtual reality simulator" in the mind. It is important to understand right at the outset that there is nothing magical or mystical about hypnosis (although hypnosis can be used in combination with spirituality). In essence, hypnosis is really a simple psychological process. All that this means is that if the brain/mind can be directed to go through the right steps, then every human being (with the exception of those with brain damage or those with severe mental handicaps) can go into hypnosis.

The fact is people go into hypnotic trances every day without being aware of it. Here are several examples of everyday hypnotic trances:

- Zoning Out

- Daydreaming

- Reading an interesting book

Those are broadly my weapons of choice. As you read on you will find that the bullets are precise and powerful. All of the following incorporate combine or use ideas from these powerful thought strategies and I would urge you to study them more via our recommendations section or find a deeper explanation in the full version of this book.

MEETING THE LADIES

I would like to introduce you to some of the 12 Fat Ladies. In this lite or e-version of the book you will meet a small selection. The whole programme has no beginning or end and as such you are welcome to use or reuse the exercise but physically trying them is essential at least once. In the full published version of the book you will find the other exercises as well as much more detail within the text. Every one of them can be of some use so my advice would be to physically try them all before deciding whether they are good or bad. Its unlikely they will all suit your pallet but most will. However before we continue, some words of caution. These tools are interesting on paper and incredible off it. Try each one at least twice. I cannot stress that enough. There are some who are not going to escape the diet cult and we may have to leave them behind. A large number of those will not go as far as actually trying these exercises at least twice. Before you actually decide to go back, try them. But first some words of caution. These weapons in the wrong hands have dangers.

GIVE UP YOUR DIET BUT DON'T GIVE UP

Giving up your diet is not your dream ticket to indulge yourself completely and abuse your body to destruction. 12 Fat Ladies is about a long term and determined goal. There is no room here for crash dieting for the wedding next month or whatever that short term goal might be. Needless to say once the pressure and preoccupation with what you eat is removed you will by default look and feel happier. As we said earlier in the book the very least you can do is be big and happy or big and unhappy but we aim to go so much further than that. Health and diet are longer term issues than just what you eat today. Lets say that I go out tonight and have a few pints and get pretty drunk. "Well what a night that was" I will say. What if I do the same the next night and the night after? One hell of a weekend maybe or even a holiday. What about a week later when I am still doing that. The week after and the week after? The point is that our health and exercise regime cannot be taken as a snapshot every single day. However your body will surely tell you when it is hungry and if its not then why eat? If it is, then why eat things that are bad for it? In the same respect do not starve it either. It might get scared and decide to store fat as soon as it gets hold of any, just in case.

ITS YOUR RESPONSIBILITY

Giving up your diet regime does not mean you are giving up responsibility for your own wellbeing it means the exact opposite. It means you are now going to take full responsibility for everything you do from this point on.

You are about to learn techniques hand-picked from the very best talk therapies. Techniques that have allowed people to be cut open without anaesthetic. Techniques that enabled me and thousands of others walk on fire without any pain or ill effects. Ways of working that I have used to reduce violence in offenders and get rid of alcohol dependency. Turn round the lives of troubled families suffering with drug abuse and violence. These therapies are lorded by success coaches, business leaders and millionaires. Its not some quick fix miracle cure but a set of useful exercises to change your beliefs about yourself and those around you and to change your identity. After that success in anything is a by product and a natural process.

12 Fat Ladies is designed to be interactive so that you will gain the knowledge and logic between each of the tools you will receive. 12 Fat Ladies is your mental gym, your food for thought. In the full printed version you will gain workable background knowledge on all the methods and models used. Knowing how something works does not stop it working. The thing to remember is that your

success will come because of small lasting changes rather than large short lived change. Like any goal its about the journey. No business man or woman ever worked through their lives imagining driving that dream car only to sit in it and say "Great I did it, I can stop work now" Because that is what they are now, its just them. Being healthier and enjoying life more without diets will become just you.

No more scales because weight is no longer relevant its about how you decide to move forward. Decide your own success based on comments or how you look in the mirror or how much happier you feel on a day to day basis.

Lets go.

EXERCISE NUMBER ONE

12 Fat Ladies ™

By Michael Dawson

QUESTION YOURSELF

Introduction

Self-task Questionnaire

"Begin with the end in mind"

The self-task questionnaire is more than just an assessment of you, it is an assessment of your mindset. It helps you start to build a picture of how you see the world and more importantly how your subconscious sees the world too. How your subconscious sees the world and your relationship to it is vital. Our mental DNA will help us settle in a comfortable safe place. It also embeds any inaccurate self-perceptions about our skills and personality as well as how we look and feel in any given situation. The beliefs embedded in your subconscious tell us where we fit in and by default it tells others. Those beliefs are more often than not unfounded and based on past experience. As human beings its natural to look for evidence to confirm those beliefs in everyday life whilst evidence to the contrary is regarded as an exception to the rule. We never question those beliefs, until now.

In any type of change it's the questions that we ask that are vital. Its just as vital to be brutally honest with yourself and that's a challenge in itself as our sessions have shown. In our sessions you are welcome to share or keep as much or as little information as you like. But in this instance be brave and honest. During my sessions with groups and individuals there have been numerous emotional moments when clients suddenly ask themselves these questions and find that the answers are not what they want. Suddenly finding out you have been selling yourself short all these years or that you are trying to achieve something that's not really for you can be uncomfortable. Realising the strengths and opportunities have been there all along and you didn't take them can be cruel. In the main though it is an uplifting experience to acknowledge your own acheivments and strengths. That's why we leave people free to decide how much they share because I would prefer you to be honest on paper and keep it to yourself than guarded with the group.

The other difficulty that arises in these situations is the mindset of the problem and the expert. The very fact that a person is receiving some kind of therapeutic input tells them they are "broken". The very fact they are seeking that input from me tells them I am the expert. Neither is true of course because only you are the expert of your own life. As a therapist I was often humbled by people who told me how they had coped for years on benefits with numerous children, an alcoholic husband and they were coming to me for help? When all they really needed was acknowledgment of their own strengths to move on. This questionnaire helps you to see what your motivations are and who they are for. After each question I have provided an explanation of what you may be hoping to see in the answers box. Clients are welcome to destroy, keep or share these at the end of the session.

I will provide a clear copy of the questionnaire further on in the book in Appendix One

Remember the power of actually writing down your answers helps to embed the thoughts and provide clarity. Its easy to just throw it away afterwards if you prefer.

What is the goal?

Make this clear, concrete and achievable. Would you know it if it tap-danced on your foot or as they say "Can you put it in a wheelbarrow" Is it real and measurable? No generalisations here like "eat less or exercise more" Make it real, measurable and specific. More importantly it should be scaled to suit you and no one else. It should be challenging and achievable. When I worked with my original group there were all sorts of different goals. I encourage you to be as imaginative as you like. This will be your benchmark to future success. One woman decided she would walk to the local shops on Saturdays instead of getting the bus. Another woman aimed to fit into a lovely pair of jeans she had never worn. One man was going to try and not buy the chocolate bar he bought every night from the train station. Incidentally every one of them achieved their goals. Not all that difficult for you maybe but to the person who sets the goal it's a giant leap forward and a great first step.

Where are you now?

In relation to the goal on a scale of 1 to 10… 1 being nothing and ten being your target where are you now? These scaling questions are very effective at providing a measure for you. It would help me to gauge where you saw yourself on a scale of one to ten. If I think 5 and you think 6 so what if I think 2 and you think 7 whatever. The important thing is you have set a clear starting point for yourself. Remember you are the expert of your own life.

What will be different when you have it?

Go to town on this one. What will you be hearing, seeing and smelling. Use all the senses in your answer. Hear the words of friends as they say "Hey your lookin good" and "I never thought you would" or "Well done how did you do it?" Can you see the faces, the new clothes or even the new job or boyfriend. Close your eyes and see those images in colour on your imaginary big screen and step into that world. You will know by now how important vivid imagery is in both a negative and positive sense. If you are fitting in that new dress feel the material comfortable against your skin and the clear bright colours.

How will you know?

What concrete signs will tell you that you have moved up ¼ point up the scale? Just one small movement towards your goal, a quarter point. Again these are mental anchors that will tell the subconscious you are making real changes. These signs have to be specific and more importantly specific to you. Walking to the shops? Maybe seeing the bus go past or feeling more tired at night. Any specific sign will confirm for you these changes are happening.

Is your goal appropriately contextualised?

What I mean is do you know where you will achieve it. Is it at home or at work? Maybe you are not going to use the lift on Fridays. So the decision is taken as to where and when you will achieve your goal. Will you need the support of others or can you do it alone? Maybe you need less support from others i.e. no lift to the shops on Saturday. A quick check to make sure that you can answer who, where, when and with whom

Is it self-initiated and self-maintained?

Is this really for you or is it for someone else? Either way it can be a motivator but its good to know. My wife wants me to lose weight or the kids. You may be perfectly happy as you are but if so can you change your behaviour for others?

Can you pretend?

Can you pretend in every way that you will achieve your target and more? We now know our internal brain has trouble working out what is true and what is real. It will build a picture from what it sees. It stores messages like trying, might do would love to and gets ready for failure. I worked with a man once who had a flying phobia and one of the key things I asked him to do between sessions was to pretend. He was an excellent client and set about his task with vigour. I asked him to tell his friends and family about his upcoming holidays, he got brochures and pictures of the aircraft. He planned his flight and hotel transfers and got prices and availability. As his little robot peeked out it could see the preparations and so it provided little resistance when finally. Three weeks later he boarded the plane to his holiday in France. So pretend and vividly prepare for your success.

The next four questions may look similar but are quite different. They will help you to weigh up the gains and losses from change. Remember the rule that every problem is usually the result of trying to solve another problem. As this happens then the problem you verbally want to rid yourself of may have underlying benefits. Smoking brings some stimulation and relaxation, bad behaviour brings attention, being needy brings support. By asking yourself the following it may become apparent that there will be losses as well as gains. Could ridding yourself of one problem bring significant gains that outweigh the losses?

What will happen if you achieve it?

What will not happen if you get it?

What will happen if you don't get it?

What will not happen if you do not get it?

When did you last come closest to achieving your goal?

Was it last week, or last year when you came closest to achieving your goal? What was different in you life then. How did that come about? Whether its weeks, days or years then there was almost certainly some pattern in your life that helped you do that. If you have read the Solution Focused Therapy Section you will know that there may well be deeper reasons that can be reproduced now

If it was someone else's goal what advice would you give to help them achieve it?

Mentally detach yourself and give some advice on how to achieve this goal and more like it. What experience do you have of past achievements and what sort of things have given you the imaginary right to advise someone like you?

If it was someone who was to have the problem for you what would you advise?

Lets suppose you could have a day off from your problem. In another world you could allow someone like me to have the problem for you whilst you had a day off. You would need to explain to me how to have our problem. I would need to know when to start eating and drinking etc and how much. Is there a signal or time to start or stop having your problem? Is there a time in the day for a rest from the problem and how do they know how to get back to it. Give me a full written run down of how to ensure your problem is still in good shape when you pick it all back up again tomorrow.

What would achieving this goal tell you about yourself?

What real lessons could you learn about yourself when you achieve this goal? Will you be surprised at your own determination and vigour? Maybe it will confirm what you have always known and it will be a stepping-stone to the next goal. More importantly you may have to redefine some of your core values and deeply held beliefs about yourself? How much fun will that be?

What resources are needed?

Do you need resources or knowledge to help you? If so what and where is it going to come from? This may be information on classes or college course, bus timetables and absolutely anything you need to get to this goal. Any physical resource.

Have you done it before or do you know someone who has?

Either way tap into that expertise either by reliving that success or asking someone else. Ask in great detail how they did it and why and how it felt. Probe, probe, probe.

Do you still want to proceed?

Well do you? Maybe after all the analysis you have realised that the goal set was too hard, too easy or just completely wide of the mark. Maybe these questions have helped you realise that its not what you want or it's the wrong time. That is your decision but if you are prepared and ready and have been completely honest with yourself then make a decision and set a date. Most importantly your goals are manageable, challenging steps that are yours and only yours.

Ensure you engage all areas of the brain by physically writing down your answers on the blank form provided in the appendix. The robot is watching and he believes you.

EXERCISE NUMBER TWO

12 Fat Ladies ™

By Michael Dawson

SWISH!

Introduction

In earlier examples I have spoken about ex-smokers who no longer spend every waking hour trying not to think about cigarettes. The reason being that cigarettes now reside in a different compartment within the brain and so there is no longer a need to avoid them. The same can be said for certain foods or habits and we have had amazing success with this exercise in our seminars. The "Swish Pattern" is another piece of brain programming developed in the world of NLP. It is an exercise that takes around 20 minutes and is incredibly powerful in changing specific low-level behaviours and attitudes. Don't worry about any of the weird stuff just try it because as with lots of these exercises you have been doing them subconsciously for years anyway.

Lets just look at your patterns of behaviour in general before the swish. Let me suggest to you that you were to consider going to the gym this evening and ask you to think what sort of emotions, images and pictures does that conjure up for you.

It may be the aggravation of having to go out of your way in the traffic, the extra effort after a long day and the sheer hard work you will have to do when you get there. The immediate attraction of the sofa and a cool glass of beer. All the reasons you feel you deserve to do something else rather than this self-inflicted chore. Stop for a moment and think. Do these kinds of images fit with your way of thinking? Don't worry if they do its perfectly normal.

Alternatively you may have very different thoughts when you think of going to the gym. The great feeling of achievement, that well deserved shower afterward and that feeling of energy and achievement. The extra buzz you get from knowing that you have improved your general physical and mental health and well-being. Maybe your first thought is of crossing the finish line of your first sports challenge whatever that might be. Again these are perfectly natural thought processes.

Remember we now know how unconsciously biased our brains are and how it seeks out confirmation of what it expects and often gets it. Once our inner beliefs change about our situation then we are bound to act differently.

The question in this situation and many more is which belief would you prefer to have and wouldn't it be great if you could switch to the more positive. That's what the swish pattern will do for you. Overcome any concerns about this on paper and try it. If you have doubts just try it on something very low key like your next team meeting and see if your attitude becomes more positive and upbeat and others follow.

It can work in all kinds of situations

- The potential anxiety before a presentation at work

- The concern over meeting a tough client

- Going to a function and meeting new people

- Preparing for an interview

The swish technique is very easy to master but first let me ask you to read to the very end of this chapter before continuing. I will run through the technique and offer some key pointers at the end. After that you just need to try it out yourself in around 15 to 20 minutes.

This book is designed as a flick through type book where you can use any or all of the techniques as and when you feel the need to. I recommend you physically road check them all in particular the ones that you think sound a bit quirky. Things are very different on paper and I have certainly been guilty myself of reading an exercise without testing it out. That being said it may be of use to look at the chapter on modalities (printed version only) although it is not essential for you to perform this exercise. Briefly though, modalities are perhaps best described as the frames of reference and they are numerous. Its true to say that when you perform this exercise it will embed better when you use a broad range of different modalities. For example if you are thinking of a bar of chocolate take the time to notice not only the appearance but the smell, taste and colour as well as any associated sounds. Use all the imaginations senses to make the picture real. Also you will find a different feeling when you see in the first person i.e. through your own eyes holding the chocolate bar instead of maybe seeing a film from a distance of you holding the chocolate bar. I am sure that makes sense and that's why you can find out more about modalities in the full version of the book.

The Swish Pattern has various stages

- Identify the issue

- Find the cue

- Choose your new response

- Swish

- Embed deeper

- Test it

THE SWISH METHOD

IDENTIFY THE ISSUE

Spend a moment thinking about what it is you would like to change about your behaviour. Is there something you would like to react to in a more positive way? It can be anything that has been suggested above or experiment with your own and see how it works but the process remains the same. For the sake of this example I am going to use a genuine example we used in our early seminars. On the face of it a relatively minor issue but one that over time had been a problem for my client. It was that whenever he got off the bus from work he would walk across the road and buy a mars bar. In itself not a big deal and in relation to his other health issues neither here nor there. As is often the case the reason he really hated it because it was confirmation of his complete lack of willpower. Those tiny failures on a daily basis served only to confirm his lack of control in other areas. This added to his stress because every day he went into the shop and paid money for another shot of self-confidence sapper. It meant a lot to him. This is the perfect anecdote for the swish because it is a relatively simple action that will have a huge mental effect. Choose your own carefully and lets say that we will attempt to change this pattern with the swish.

FIND THE CUE

The next task is to find the cue that instigates the behaviour. What is the trigger or stimulus that sets your actions in motion? If this is a problem then a good idea is to imagine you were having a day off and you have to leave instructions for a stranger to do this for you. The instructions will have to be concise and clear. Is it when you get up out of your seat to get off the bus, are you checking your change to make sure you have the cash. Maybe its hours earlier when you buy lunch that you place your 48p to one side. Walking down the road and seeing the news sign or the smell of the bus pulling away. Run through your own scenario in your head and see it as a film with you being the first person. It can often help to take a still Polaroid in our head too. In this case it was in fact checking his change before he got off the bus. The powerful still image i.e. the last thing he saw before his brain pulled the trigger was in fact the bell to stop the bus. Hold that thought and clear your mind completely. See how many trees you can see out of the window or think of your phone number. This just helps to reset your brain.

CHOOSE YOUR NEW RESPONSE

You will need to decide what you want to replace this behaviour with but in most cases if you want to avoid a habit that just means nothing. Our brain is not so keen on being motivated by nothing and in fact it does not have to be a physical action. It can be the result that you want to attach to the swish. In the case of the Mars bar it was a clear crisp image of the new you. His new self-image which involved as many modalities as he could fit into it. He saw himself looking and feeling fitter and wearing the clothes he would be buying. He heard the voices of congratulation and adulation for his achievements. He saw this in vibrant bright colours and it was there in front of him and he could see it and be in it too. Then just for good measure he took the snapshot as a memento. It is important that you view yourself from a distance. This will become clearer later. Now he had all the elements he needed to perform the swish.

NOW SWISH!

The swish can be performed anywhere that you can sit undisturbed for about twenty minutes. It will take you twenty minutes to do this and the effect could be dramatic. Take image one which is the negative image and place that right in front of your minds eye. When you can see it nice and clearly take the second image, the positive one and cover it over. Next take the positive image and push it up into the corner as a tiny thumbnail. What you will do next is attach imaginary elastic bands to both images. The positive image will be attached to some point behind you and the negative to some point in the distance. Remember this is all in your minds eye so make it big and bold. You could attach one image to the moon and one to Australia. What you are going to do next is release the images so that the positive image comes crashing through the negative one. Pow right there in front of you clear and crisp and bright. Visualise the image and then place them back in their positions.

Embed deeper

This time pull the negative image as far as the moon so it's a ting spec and let go. Pow! This time it comes crashing through even bigger and brighter shattering the old image.

Now your getting the idea. Never pull the negative back into view by the way that just appears. Your positive one is stretched further and further back until it's a tiny spec and Pow. This is the format and the power of this image crashing through the old will become clearer and more powerful.

Continue this routine for around ten times and then relax and empty your mind in the usual way

Test it

The next thing to do is to test the old stimulus to see if it has the same effect or feeling. To see if you get the same urges or it has the same power. Our client did just that and returned to our seminar after a week to say that after buying a Mars bar every day for as long as he can remember he had not done so on the Monday at all. This was incredible to him, even more so when you consider he didn't do it on the Tuesday or for the rest of the week! This small step was a massive boost to his self-confidence and the negative trigger became weaker and weaker.

Ok if this is your first read through then you are almost ready to give it a go but first let me give you a few pointers to make this pattern as powerful as it can be for you

Congruence of change

Another lesson we have probably learned by now in reading this book is that we can easily fool our little man or subconscious but we have deep embedded standards. Your subconscious will only operate within its own standards and goals. Hence you cannot hypnotise someone to do something they would not do consciously. So keep it real

Picture associate

Run through your colourful film, sound, small and any other powerful modalities but remember to see it all. Vision is a powerful medium for the brain to work with.

Go through the modalities

Use all the different modalities to develop the vision of the behaviour you want to develop and adapt to. Although this is a visual exercise your brain will attach all these things to that image.

The trigger

When trying to find the trigger it often helps to not think too deeply about it. As soon as you think of the association then your subconscious knows exactly what the trigger is because it has been acting on it for so long. If its not too keen to reveal that information then of course you can run through a problem lesson and just explain in detail to a stranger how they could have this problem for you.

Make the new state bigger than the unwanted state

Make your positive state bigger and louder and crystal clear by comparison to the existing negative state. You want to dwarf the old state so that it sends a clear message to our unconscious like a distracting flag being waved. "Hey never mind that look at this"

Disassociate the new state

When you run your image or movie for the new state then make sure you are watching on. If you see yourself picking up the award for the greatest speech ever then watch it on the screen as opposed to through your own eyes. The brain has to know it is seeing the future and that's where its heading.

Make the swish fast and furious

The swish should be fast, loud and furious. The old state merely opens up in front of your eyes. See the new state pull back into the distance and come crashing through like a tank through a shop window sending the old image shattering into tiny pieces.

In the coming week

Now you have installed a swish pattern that is quickly testable. If so and it works then great. Remember you can keep it topped up at any time and maybe if you are facing the challenge tomorrow then you should be prepared and run through the swish technique the night before. Run through your successes through the week so that you can evaluate your progress. Remember that changing these behaviours tends to become permanent and unconscious. There are only so many times you can make brilliant presentations before you have to accept. "I am just good at that "

EXERCISE NUMBER FIVE

12 Fat Ladies ™

By Michael Dawson

THEATRE OF DREAMS

Introduction

SELF-VISUALISATION

This book is designed to be very simple to use, no need for any in depth reading if you don't want to. If you want more background to the methods used then by all means find it here in this book and in the suggested reading section. In the meantime flick through and try something new. However because of the nature of the next exercise I recommend you look at the full printed version for some background should you need reassurance. Not because there is any danger from visualization because we all do it every day anyway as we daydream about our holiday or that new promotion you fancy. Unlike the other exercises I just believe it will work better for you with a little knowledge. The fear and mystery surrounding hypnosis and visualization is harboured and encouraged by people like me. It helps us to increase confidence and sell the method but in the end it just works anyway. But still at the very least do read through this entire section before beginning.

The theory of the subconscious is a huge and complex subject but a good metaphor might be the little robot as in the poem earlier. The subconscious wants what is best for us at all times. He holds the controls to lots of our physical and mental make-up from fight or flight to Me-n-a. He is deep in the control room and protects us even whilst we are asleep. The problem is that despite this he often gets things wrong. He has no language and so you cannot tell him things. He receives messages from the conscious in the form of analogies and generalisations, its easier that way. He peeks through a tiny porthole and can often make very broad assumptions about us and his decisions seem very bizarre. If bad things happen to us he never wants that to happen again and so will pick out patterns and avoid them. If you fail at something he may interpret that as it being safer to avoid trying again in the future. He is always on call and always paying attention. Using the same metaphor we can use hypnosis to distract him and so kind of download experiences and messages. He will accept most of them as real and adjust the controls accordingly. He has a very good filter though and for some reason he will reject messages that clash with our higher moral standing. In a weird way he would be happy to run around pretending to be a chicken but to genuinely hurt someone would not get through the filter. He also picks up information about us from our conscious thoughts. He is not very good at determining what is real and what fantasy is. That's why we feel angry when we remember an argument or hostility to certain types of people without justification. Its also true that he does not understand negatives very well. If you say "I must not eat that" or "I must not think that" then he has to think it to not think it. This can cause problems for us all in particular this raises problems with diet behaviour which insists we focus on calories and foods etc. The evidence and studies from Wegner show that this can produce an obsession about the very thing we want to avoid. The good news is that once we understand the little robot he will work very well for us. He will interpret our positive messages and help us to act accordingly. Of course all of the above is to help us understand and despite all the theory on though, understanding and hypnosis there are none which are conclusive. It just helps to think of it in this way as long as it works. When hypnosis works it is often invisible. Quite often there is a feeling of

"Yeh I tried that Hypnosis thing but in the end I just did it myself"

As we say in other therapies it is perfect in that sometimes it leaves no footprints. More often even the actual act of hypnosis becomes invisible too. This is probably best illustrated by a true story of when I was training with the London School of Hypnotherapy and we were in our sixth week on the course. By this time we were grasping the model to a point where we were able to have discussions privately about the methods used. It was over lunch with a couple of my fellow students that I happened to mention how things had moved on from our very first day. On our very first day we had been hypnotized as a group and had been told a story about a ship going on a voyage. During the trance the teacher had spoken about being sea worthy and ready for a long and fruitful journey. I could still see my own personal ship in my mind and the shiny polished brass rails and crisp strong sails etc. It was still a vivid memory created by myself.

One of the guys interrupts me "What ship, there was no story on the first day about any ship"

"Of course there was" I said looking around for confirmation and all I got was blank stares from the four people sat around the table.

"Does no one remember the story of the ship?"

I was convinced there had been a visualization story about a ship preparing to go on a long journey but maybe I had created my own personal story. We then went back to the class of which there were about 30 students and asked pretty much everyone. To my surprise there were another three people in the whole class who said quite matter of fact. "oh that yeh, the ship and everything" Just as I had described it. It did happen but only about 5/8% of the class had any conscious memory of it at all. Either most of the class were much deeper than us or maybe their subconscious minds realized that they had no real need to remember the method, just the message. Another example of the lack of footprints is what happened to me when I worked on my fear of flying. I consciously knew I was afraid of flying. That was me and had been for a long time and so when I got to the airport I had decided to go ahead. I was not as afraid as usual and by the time I got off the plane I had a feeling of how quick it had gone but it just was not as bad as usual. That's when it hits you in my experience. You don't always experience the change whilst its happening but the signposts will confirm your movement forward. All of a sudden I had gone through what would normally have been a very unpleasant experience without recognizing it.

The second part of hypnosis that can be invisible is what I call signposts. This is where you do a session of self-hypnosis and you are never quite sure if it has made a difference until you hit a sign post. That is a point in your change where you realize you are behaving differently. A clever practitioner will always put sign posts in place along the journey of change. In this case the practitioner will be yourself. A sign post is most likely to be a symptom of the change that will happen anyway whether negative or positive. An example might be in giving up smoking. It may be the familiar cravings; these will be set up merely to serve as a reminder that you are making progress and are moving towards your goal.

On to the method, firstly of course I would suggest browsing the hypnosis section in the printed version if you have it, this is not essential but certainly read through this entire section before practicing. It goes without saying that allthough this is not hypnosis in the truest sense of the word be cautious if you have any kind of mental health diagnosis.

SETTING GOALS

Firstly it's important to set the goals of the session before you start. If you have done exercise two and completed the questionnaire fully you should now have a crystal clear idea in your mind of where you are going and why. If you haven't then now would be a really good time to explore that because it will be a huge help with everything else you do. Remember that the goals you set for yourself in a hypnosis session should be in the positive. Therefore I want to have more self-control is much better than I want to stop eating X Y or Z. It's also important to trust your subconscious and allow it to guide you through the process. There are lots of self-visualization methods and millions of scripts and our seminars are not designed to make you a skilled hypnotherapist. I will guide you through a single session and you will improve with practice.

WRITING YOUR SCRIPT

The next stage is to write your script and read through it. I have provided some example scripts for you in appendix two but you would be advised to revise them to suit yourself. You do not have to memorise the script just be very familiar with its story. This can be done in a number of ways. The main thing to remember is not to clash with your subconscious but to work with it. That means that your visualization process should be in terms that are familiar to you and that you are comfortable with. Our minds are quite happy with the concept of down relating to relaxation. During the deepener you can use numbers, stairs or even your own physical self by relaxing from top to bottom. As you become advanced you may learn to add a second deepener so once you reach one then you start from ten again and work down once more. During the actual visualization stage then again its worth using familiar territory that does not clash with your subconscious. I once had a client who was distracted by being in a wonderful calm woods watching a TV screen but could not work out how to plug it in! A fair point I suppose so we had to change his location to his own bedroom which served the purpose perfectly because it is a place of safety for him.

IMAGINE YOUR SUCCESS

As an example lets try something fairly straightforward and adaptable. The full script is in appendix two but heres how it works

At the bottom of your deepener you are going to find there are a series of doors. Above the doors is a sign that says "Your Success"

Printed on each door is a time period as follows

- Door 1   1 Week

- Door 2   1 Month

- Door 3   6 Months

- Door 4   1 Year

- Door 5   5 Years

- Door 6   10 years

Behind every door will be your personal realized future. This exercise will also act as a sign post as discussed later. When you have decided which door to go through you will be able to experience the success you have achieved and experience how that feels. Importantly immerse yourself in the experience using every sense. Hear the voices of congratulations, the sound of applause and any other elated sounds. See in vivid colour where you are, how you look and how everyone, even the smells and aromas are used to enhance the experience you are about to have. Once you are ready you can then leave by the door you came in and beginning your count out of hypnosis

You will already have decided how long your entire session will be before starting and have read your script carefully. Whilst in your relaxed state the actual words of the script are not important as long as you have a good idea of what you will be achieving.

Choose a place of comfort to do your session and sitting in an upright position without crossing legs or arms is suggested. If you can expect to be undisturbed then that would be a great advantage. You will by now be aware from the questions section that you cannot get stuck in trance. If the fire alarm goes off or the door goes then you will simply open your eyes, orientate yourself for a moment and leave the session. You always have the choice to ignore distractions like the binmen arriving or a dog barking. You simply tell yourself in similar words. "I can choose to ignore the sound of if I wish and focus on my own voice" As with a lot of hypnosis and visualization it will make a lot more sense when you experience it than in the written word. Some light relaxing music either from your own CD collection or from the many on sale will be of greater benefit throughout.

AWAKENING

The scripts you will find in this book and around the web are similar in nature but you should notice the common use of words and suggestion. Sitting reading the scripts does tend to sound odd but in a hypnotic trance they do not. Hopefully you will have proved that self-hypnosis is just as effective in helping you with numerous problems.

When personalizing your script or story for visualization remember to use familiar and comfortable places and settings. Also use language that you feel natural with and allow yourself to use all the senses such as visual, auditory and touch. The more natural and comfortable the messenger the less resistance your subconscious will come up against.

There are some example scripts here and lots on the internet to choose from and use. Pretty much every one of them will sound silly when read out but don't let that put you off trying to give it a go.

WHAT HAVE WE LEARNED?

We are now safely over the wall and are having to adapt to a new environment. There will be ex diet converts who want to bring you back, there will be concerned family members who have never known you not diet. They will worry that you will binge or fall backwards without knowing that you are now in control not the robot. For you there will be occasions when you start to feel like one of the weightless people and as such share their eating habits. There are no scales to weigh yourself but you don't need them anymore. Everything is about how you feel and look. The benefits tend to come in chunks so don't worry or fuss about it. It was just one of those things you or other people notice occasionally.

There will be changes that stay forever so you have all the time in the world to let your body know it will have food when it needs it and it has no need to crash diet. In time the changes however small will just be normal, they are just what you do.

Hopefully you will continue to read or study some of the suggested material or even look up the full printed version of this book which contains more exercises and all the background information about the therapies. There is also a comprehensive rules of engagement section which applies to all levels of your life.

12 Fat Ladies was adapted for weight control and healthy living but contains nothing about nutrition or diet. That's because it does not need to and the same rules apply no matter what you want to do. These exercises will help you at work,

with family and relationships or any form of challenge as long as you physically do them.

If you have done these exercises or discovered your own please remember I always love to hear from readers. Comment on our blog and forum at www.12fatladies.com or come and say hello at one of my seminars

ACKNOWLEDGEMENTS AND FURTHER READING

This book would never have been possible without the fantastic work of those who came before me. I have read and studied a million books on the subject and will miss out countless acknowledgments but I am indebted to you just the same. I also want to thank the hard work and dedication of numerous clients I have worked with who have taught me so many lessons. The names, titles and studies below are a fraction of the recommended reading and major influence of this book.

My voice will go with you by Sidney Rosen - Norton Publishing

The Luck Factor by Dr Richard Wiseman - Century Publishing

Understanding Neuro Linguistic Programming in a week by Mo Shapiro - Hodder and Stoughton

Bring Out the Magic in your Mind by A Koran - A Thomas Publishing

Use your Head by Tony Buzan - BBC Publishing

Self Hypnosis by Dr Brian L Alman & Dr Peter Lambrou

The Mind Gym - Time Warner Books

Problem to Solution by Evan George Chris Iverson and HArvey Ratner - BT Press

12 Fat Ladies (Full Text) will be published March 2012

For the latest weblinks and exercises then register with our blog at www.12fatladies.com

APPENDIX 1

EXERCISE NUMBER ONE

12 Fat Ladies ™

By Michael Dawson

QUESTION YOURSELF

What is the goal?

Where are you now?

What will be different when you have it?

How will you know?

Is your goal appropriately contextualised?

Is it self-initiated and self-maintained?

Can you pretend?

What will happen if you achieve it?

What will not happen if you get it?

What will happen if you don't get it?

What will not happen if you do not get it?

When did you last come closest to achieving your goal?

If it was someone else's goal what advice would you give to help them achieve it?

If it was someone was to have the problem for you what would you advise?

What would achieving this goal tell you about yourself?

What resources are needed?

Have you done it before or do you know someone who has?

Do you still want to proceed?

APPENDIX 2

HYPNOTIC INDUCTION SCRIPT

The following can be recorded by you and replayed with headphones

Make yourself comfortable and sit upright with feet flat on the floor and your hands on your lap.

When your ready you can allow your eyes to close........and feel yourself relax......for a short time you can allow any cares or worries to drift away....................at this moment nothing else is of significance.........you can switch off your thoughts.......allowing this time for yourself..........you can rewind completely.......and as you begin to feel more and more relaxed.........you can unwind completely.......there is no need to fight any negative thoughts or feelings.......they will naturally drift away........they will drift away.....as easily and naturally as they came....i would like you to become focused on my voice......as you do you can breathe in deeply and breath out slowly relaxing as you do with each breath.....you can become more and more aware of your breathing.....aware of relaxing deeper and deeper with every breath...........more and more relaxed.......more and more comfortable......you may notice your whole body....sinking....deeper....and deeper into that comfortable state of relaxation....completely relaxed from the top of your head.....to the tips of your toes......your eyelids will feel heavier....the small muscles in your face become relaxed.....completely at ease.....completely natural....as if floating.....the last of the tension flowing out of your body....you may feel more and more relaxed with every word I speak...   more and....more...its natural for the feeling of relaxation to travel down your body....down your neck and arms....and your arms become as heavy as lead.....you will feel completely at peace now.....your chest and abdomen relaxed....your back warm and relaxed...perfectly calm and natural.....deeper and deeper...you can let the wave of relaxation travel down to your legs and feet....noticing how you are completely relaxed from the top of your head to the tips of your toes....the outside world is now just in the background...as you choose to concentrate only on my voice....just my words.... Your limbs heavy as lead....warm relaxed drifting comfortably...you will feel ready now to relax and let the world drift into the background.....its easy now to ignore any negative thoughts or feelings.....easy to ignore any sounds close or in the distance......the sound of my voice will help you go deeper....and deeper...into a wonderful state of relaxation.........on a journey into a special part of you.....where only you can go.....safe ...secure...relaxed...you may find that your mind begins to wonder....that will not matter...my voice will go with you....you can choose to focus on my voice....it will stay with you...and you will still respond on an unconscious level...in a few moments time you will hear me begin to count....down from ten to one....as I count you will become more and more relaxed....sinking deeper and deeper......with every count down....you will be another level more relaxed....another level less tension....you will enjoy this wonderful feeling of relaxation more....and more with every level...ready...ten...deeper and deeper relaxed.....nine...limbs becoming heavy like lead.....heavy and limp.....as you become deeper and deeper relaxed you may drift away...eight.... This is perfectly natural...seven...deeper....six...more and more relaxed.......five....heavy as lead....four.....deeper and deeper...drifting away....three....natural relaxing.....two.....deeper and deeper and one...completely relaxed now....floating and comfortable..and now in a few moments time...you can allow your mind to enjoy a journey...to a place deep inside your mind....and my voice will guide you.

©mdawson2010

HYPNOTIC VISUALISATION SCRIPT

The following can be recorded by you and replayed with headphones

And now... as you continue to drift....in this relaxed state of mind....i want you to know something about being in this state....in this trance state you can do anything you want to....safely.....and securely...like a pleasant dream......you are able to drift away with your inner mind...to places in the past and places in the future...real places and imaginary places....any situation you desire....you can experience.....you can vist places special to you....these are the wonderful things about being so relaxed...in a dream you can control...

Whilst my voice will always go with you....my voice will guide you....and soon I will ask you to imagine a place...,somewhere you have never been.....somewhere you wish to be...where you are safe and relaxed....very soon you will imagine going there.....very soon you will be in that place.....and now you are there...enjoying the experience...whilst here you can relax a little deeper if you wish...comfortable and relaxed....its in this place that you will find a wonderful experience...an experience unique only to you and your inner mind....but so vivid and real..here...now...whilst looking around you will notice....there are six doors.,..six doors created by you....and behind each door is an experience....an experience of your imagined future...each door has a sign on it.....the first door says 6 months from now.....the second one year from now....the third 2 years...the fourth 3 years....the fifth door 5 years... and door six just a question mark....very soon I am going to ask you to pick a door....all the doors contain a wonderful experience from your future.....every door is going to allow you to experience something good...and now..i am going to ask you to choose a door...as you approach that door...you can turn the handle....and it almost opens on its own...as light as air...and as you step through you will find yourself there......in that place....here you can enjoy the feelings you have at that time.....powerful....confident....stronger...able to make those decisions....you will see and feel your success....you may be able to hear the voices of those around you......it's a euphoric feeling of control and feeling powerful.......this experience is unique just to you only....in your own mind......there may even be other sensations....there may even be other memories of how you arrived at this future....the challenges you overcame....only you will know...you can enjoy this experience for a moment......relax and absorb the feeling......I want you to know that.......whilst in this state you can fully enjoy the experience......and soon you will leave this place.....soon I will ask you to leave.....but should you choose...you can take this feeling with you......you can return knowing.....your chosen future is possible....if you want that....you can feel it here...you can see it here...and those memories will be like stepping stones.....each challenge overcome will be another step towards.....your imagined future.....you will recognise those steps as you travel along the way....as you day by day.....week by week...month by month....become stronger.....more confident.....able to make clearer decisions.....moving powerfully and determined towards your goals....and now I am going to ask you to find the door....to walk back through to your imagined place.....you will know you can return....you can return anytime.....in your own mind......your deep unconscious mind will know the path.....will know you are stronger.....more determined day by day....every day.....

©mdawson2010

HYPNOTIC AWAKENING SCRIPT

The following can be recorded by you and replayed with headphones

And very soon now....i am going to wake you.......but before I do........i would like you to know that as each day goes by.....you are going to feel more in control....which means you are going to be able to think more clearly........so much so that soon no one.....or no situation will be able to worry you.....you will feel this as every day goes by............and as the days......weeks....months go by you will fel calmer....more relaxed....more in control........a greater feeling of well-being........a greater feeling of satisfaction with your life.......in a few moments I am going to wake you......i am going start to count......one to ten.....with every number you will become more awake.....more alert......by the count of eight you will open your eyes and by the count of ten you will be wide awake........you will be awake with a feeling of well-being all over.......with every part of you refreshed and back here with me in the present......so.....ready.....one......two......waking......three.......four....waking... .....waking....five.......six......seven....more awake........eight....open your eyes....nine....ten.....wide awake....wide awake....back here in the room with me

©mdawson2010

About the author

Michael has spent over twenty years in the field working for the mental health service, family therapy and in clinical hypnosis. Along the way he has studied and used many different models of working from Neuro Linguistic Programming to Solution Focused Brief Therapy and Hypnosis. Over time he developed his own dynamic methods from the best of the best. He has trained a wide range of professionals in talking therapies over the years including Police, Mental health and social workers as well as teachers and social workers.

He is an experienced training provider and speaker based in the North West of England.

He is the author of the revolutionary 12 Fat Ladies ™ programme designed to free individuals from the diet trap forever.

CONTACT

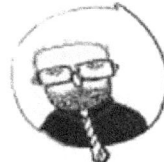 Michael is available on occasion for interview and speaking engagements regarding the 12 Fat Ladies Programme. Clients are also most welcome to email or comment either directly or through the website.

www.12fatladies.com   info@12fatladies.com

www.ingramcontent.com/pod-product-compliance
Lightning Source LLC
Chambersburg PA
CBHW081832280526

45789CB00007B/2429